Healthy Living

How To Take Care Of Your Body

Chapter 1 *living a healthy lifestyle*

Water is by far the most important resource in the world, yet it garners the respect of so few. How often do you find yourself standing with the fridge door open looking for something to drink – completely ignoring your jug of filtered water that sits before your eyes?

Knees hurt? Do this once daily and watch what happens

The truth is, water should always be the beverage of choice. While the human body can go about 3 weeks without food, it cannot survive for more than 3 days without water.

Water is essential to every bodily function. No other liquid can sustain your body like water, and the body needs a certain amount of water to function well.

About 80% of the human brain is water, blood contains 83% water, the lungs 79% and muscles 76%. All in all, the human body is about 75% water. Every function in the body is dependent on a steady supply and flow of water.

Water transports such things as hormones, chemicals and nutrients which are vital to efficient organ function. Without water we would not be able to digest or absorb minerals or nutrients and our kidneys would fail from toxic overload.

Water is, in fact, a sort of miracle elixir – but have you ever thought of it that way?

Here are just a few of the amazing things that water can do for your health:

keep skin vibrant and supple
escort toxins from the body

support healthy metabolism
improve energy
remove body heat
lubricate joints
improve mental and physical performance
support digestion
But hold on… we are just getting started. Water, yes, simple, plain old water, the same water that you might bypass for something more glamourous… not only sustains life but holds within it the capacity to heal. Here are sixteen illnesses that water can help prevent and reverse. We hope that after reading this article you will be convinced that water should ALWAYS be your first beverage of choice.

Arthritis

It is estimated that over 52 million adults in the United States have some form of arthritis – which literally means "joint inflammation". The pain and discomfort of this condition varies from a minor inconvenience to a full-blown disability. Millions of dollars are spent on anti-inflammatory and pain medications that often have harsh side effects.

Persons suffering from arthritis are often subjected to a life sentence to these harsh drugs, but there may be a better way. The most important thing that someone with arthritis can do is to make sure that their joints are lubricated, and water can do this. Water not only lubricates but also pads joints and reduces the friction that causes pain.

A suction-like motion pulls water from bone marrow to the joint cavity; this helps joints glide easily. If there is not enough water available it causes friction and eventually pain. If you are severely dehydrated, dry cartilage can die and peel off from the contact surface of the bones.

Gout

Gout, being a form of arthritis, is also markedly improved if not completed kept at bay with a proper consumption of water. Water helps to remove uric acid and other toxins from joints that build-up causing swelling and pain.

Osteoporosis

This painful condition is characterized by low bone mass and a structural breaking down of bone tissue. Over 10 million Americans suffer from osteoporosis and over 34 million have low bone mass – a precursor to this disease. Although there are certain risk factors that are out of our control, such as race and gender, there is much that we can control – such as how much water we consume. Water not only helps prevent this condition but it can also help sufferers cope.

Heart Disease

Often called the silent killer, taking the lives of almost 2,200 people daily – yes, we said daily. Heart disease is rampant and we seem to be able to do little to control it. However, it appears as though there is a strong relationship between water and coronary health. One study demonstrated that drinking 5 or more glasses of water per day can cut the risk of dying from a heart attack by 50%. Study leaders say that drinking water is as important as exercising, not smoking and diet in preventing heart disease.

Constipation

Constipation is an annoying and often painful condition that millions of Americans suffer from. If you have less than 3 stools per week you are constipated. If you have less than one stool a week, you are severely constipated.

The cause of constipation can be traced back to any number of things, including poor diet, medication, poor bowel habits, dehydration, hormonal disorders and laxative abuse. For many people, the discomfort of constipation becomes so great that they reach for over-the-counter medications for relief. Unfortunately, many of these medications only mask the symptoms and can make the problem worse.

It is important to consume a diet that contains healthy fats, fibers, vitamins and minerals, but it is equally important to consume adequate amounts of water. Not only does water help rid the body of toxins but it also supports healthy digestion. When you are hydrated, less water will be taken from the colon – leaving stools softer and easier to pass.

Hypertension

Many people have high blood pressure and don't even know it. Of course such things as dropping a few pounds, adopting a healthy diet and exercising can all help keep blood pressure in its normal ranges – but did you know how important it is to drink water as well?

When you don't consume enough water the body actually hangs on to sodium to preserve fluids. Dehydration forces the shutdown of capillary beds and puts a tremendous pressure on both capillaries and arteries which elevates blood pressure. So, staying well-hydrated is a very important part of keeping hypertension at bay.

Fever

Starve a fever – feed a cold, is a common saying we hear a lot. What about hydrate a fever instead? Having a fever actually means that the body is fighting off an illness or an infection and is a good sign that things aren't quite right. Having a fever leads to dehydration because the body will drain water from cells. Fever causes fluid loss and it is paramount that you replace these fluids – water is the best choice. Dehydration can make symptoms worse and cause additional discomfort.

Skin Issues

You may not think about your skin as an organ but in fact, it is the body's largest organ and is comprised of cells that are made up of water. Just like any other organ, skin needs water to be healthy. Many skin conditions such as overly dry, flaky or blotchy skin may be the result of dehydration. Without adequate water, skin can age prematurely and develop a greater number of wrinkles.

Sleep Disturbances

One in three persons suffer from some kind of sleep disturbance, more commonly known as insomnia. Characterized by a persistent problem falling asleep or staying asleep, insomnia can interfere with your work and social life and also contribute to serious health conditions.

An alarming number of people turn to both prescription and over-the-counter sleeping pills to ease their suffering. However, these pills are dangerous and can be highly addictive. Like so many other conditions, an adequate water intake is essential to reducing overall inflammation which can interfere with a good night's sleep. When combined with a healthy diet, stress management and exercise, it is possible to develop a healthy sleeping routine without the use of medication.

Yeast Infection

Yeast infections, caused by a fungus, are annoying and can be very painful. Almost 75% of women will be impacted by one of these infections in their lifetime – some more than others. Although many people turn to garlic and yogurt to combat these infections, one of the best tools is actually pure and simple water.

The more water you drink, the more you flush out excess sugars that can cause yeast infections. If you are prone to yeast infections, adding plenty of water to a healthy diet along with managing stress can prove to be one of the most effective tools for keeping infections at bay.

Colds

According to the National Institute of Allergy and Infectious Diseases in Bethesda, MD., Americans suffer over one billion colds each year. Oh the dreaded cold; runny nose, sore throat, lack of energy and the host of other uncomfortable symptoms that go with it drag so many people down.

Over-the-counter drugs only seem to keep symptoms at bay – and some, don't do this very well. The truth be known, once you get a cold virus there is very little you can do but ride it out as comfortably as possible.

However, you can do things to keep a cold from turning your life upside down in the first place – including washing hands and eating a healthy diet. While you may do these things, it is easy to forget that one of the best ways to keep yourself healthy is to replace lost fluids with water. Water helps to flush out toxins and also helps the body to produce mucus. When fighting off a cold, the body needs more water than usual and can easily get dehydrated.

Blood Sugar

According to French researchers, drinking four or more 8 ounce glasses of water per day can prevent the development of high blood sugar – a condition known as prediabetes. One in three Americans have this dangerous precursor to diabetes.

Researchers state that a hormone called vasopressin (an antidiuretic hormone) helps to balance water retention. When we become dehydrated, the levels of this hormone increase which causes the kidneys to conserve water. Studies indicate that there are vasopressin receptors in the liver – which produces glucose in the body and that higher levels of vasopressin may cause a rise in blood sugar.

Bladder Infection

Although the bladder passes fluids from the body – it needs water to do its job. The elastic muscle fibers of the bladder allow it to expand and store up to 750 ml of fluid. Pressure on the bladder walls trigger the need to urinate. Bladder infections are the result of bacteria entering the urine, which in turn creates the same urge to urinate as a full bladder. Consuming 6-8 glasses of water each day can help keep the bladder healthy and free from bacteria.

The Healing Power Of Water:

Kidney Stones

A proper supply of water helps to keep the kidneys functioning properly. Kidneys, along with the liver and urinary tract, are responsible for ridding the body of toxic materials. If the kidneys stop doing its job for just two days, metabolic toxins would accumulate and cause poisoning. When bacteria and proteins build up, stones (crystals) form – these are very painful and can be difficult to pass. Studies indicate that dehydration can increase the chance of stones to develop.

Asthma and Seasonal Allergies

According to studies, a lack of water vapor in the lungs can cause airways to constrict and produce mucus – this can bring on an asthma attack. For this reason it is vital that persons suffering with asthma drink plenty of water each day. At least ten 8 ounce glasses are recommended.

If you suffer from seasonal allergies, it is also highly important to stay hydrated. Drinking water helps the body flush out irritants, thins mucus and helps with sinus drainage.

What kind of water should I drink?

There are some people who drink enough water but are not consuming the right water. Perhaps you are under the assumption that your tap water is safe because the government says it is safe? In fact, your tap water might contain up to 80 so called "regulated" contaminants and many unregulated toxins.

Perhaps you purchase bottled water in an attempt to stay safe, however, there is a major problem with deceptive labelling in the bottled water industry.

Don't be fooled by marketing campaigns that state that the water is from a spring or pristine pool. Bottled water is just water and a very, very big business. Each year, over $75 billion dollars are spent on bottled water.

Bottled water in the United States falls under the authority of the FDA. Since over 70% of bottled water never crosses a state line for sale, it is exempt from the scrutiny of the FDA.
Tests done on bottled water have turned up traces of carcinogenic compounds, pharmaceuticals, fluoride, and arsenic to name a few. Bottled

water is not a good value and creates mounds and mounds of trash that ends up in our oceans and landfills, no matter how much we recycle.

Toxins in Drinking Water

Fluoride

Known as an extremely dangerous toxin, fluoride is added to water sources including municipal water as well as bottled water. Adding fluoride to water has been banned in other countries but remains a common practice in many American cities; although some have rejected this practice since as early as 1990.

Arsenic

Arsenic is a heavy, toxic metal that is classified by the International Academy for Research on Cancer as a Category 1 carcinogen. This means that it is a known cancer causing metal. The Environmental Protection Agency set the acceptable standard for arsenic at 10 parts per billion in tap water. Many states exceed this standard.

Chlorine

Inhaling chlorine is dangerous to health and ingesting it is even more so. Chlorine is added to water to kill certain bacteria. Once chlorine enters the body, it joins with other compounds to form Trihalomethanes which trigger free radical damage. In a recent study, chlorine was added to the water supply of rats who developed tumors in their intestines, liver and kidneys.

The United States Council of Environmental Quality, states that people who consume water with chlorine have an over 90% higher risk of developing cancer than those who don't. Even after the results of this and other similar studies have been presented before the government, chlorine continues to be added to water.

Options

So, after reading this you may be thinking, what should I drink if I cannot drink tap or bottled water? Here are a few options; as with anything, be sure that these options are suitable for your needs and do your research before making a purchase. Some systems are better than others at removing harmful contaminants. Arrange to have your tap water tested so that you know what it is you need to filter out.

There are a few options to consider when it comes to improving the quality of your drinking water. A whole house water filtration system may set you back a few bucks, but it is worth it in the long run. A good system will filter multiple impurities including chlorine from your entire water supply and requires only minor maintenance like changing the filter.

Reverse osmosis systems, either countertop, under the counter or whole house types can be costly and actually strip water of just about everything, including healthy trace minerals. Do not use a reverse osmosis filter system unless you are going to supplement your diet with trace minerals. Pitcher filtration systems that go in the refrigerator are inexpensive, but many often fall short of removing all water contaminants. However, we have found one type of pitcher filtration system that actually does work and leaves the water tasting amazing.

How much water should I drink?

If your urine has low odor and is pale colored, you are most likely on track. Some health practitioners say to aim for at least ten glasses a day, while others recommend half of your body weight in ounces.

Of course, if you are working out or spending time outdoors in the heat, it is essential that you replace water lost due to perspiration. You can also pull the skin on the top of your hand to see if it bounces back. If it stays up for a while, grab a glass or two of water, your tank is probably low.

So, it is clear, the next time you really want something to drink – push the soda, fruity juice concoctions, energy drinks, etc. aside and satisfy yourself with pure and natural water – your body will thank you.

The Meat Diet: Better than Vegetarian for Fat Loss, Diabetes, Autoimmune Issues, Digestion and More...

You may have heard in the news in the last couple years that "carnivore diets" have been growing in popularity, and have some surprisingly powerful health benefits that often shock a lot of people, since this way of eating is so contrary to what you hear in the mass media.

In fact, you may have even heard that the famous Joe Rogan (comedian and most popular podcast host in the world) tried a full month of a carnivore diet in 2020 and said it was the "best he's ever felt" while also losing 12 lbs of body fat and losing his love handles that he could never get rid of previously. He also reported that his energy was perfectly stable for the month that he ate carnivore. He felt so good eating an all-meat diet that he did it for 30 days again this past January, and reported similar results again.

As you read today's newsletter, I'd encourage you to be open minded and realize that most "gurus" out there that you hear from in the media actually don't have much depth of nutrition education, and most powerful food companies that sell ultra-processed "plant based" junk food actually have a lot of influence on spreading propaganda trying to blame all health problems on meat, eggs, and other healthy animal foods because they know that you'll buy more highly profitable "plant-based" junk food if you eat less animal food.

But when you dig into the real science, and explore it with an open mind, you actually find that most information about nutrition that's preached in the mainstream isn't necessarily correct, and I'll explain some of my findings in this email.

If you've never heard of the "carnivore diet", it's basically a way of eating that focuses either entirely or mostly on healthy meat, fish, and eggs, while avoiding most plant-foods, or choosing only small amounts of plant foods based on a scale of plant toxicity... for example, with leafy greens, nightshades, grains, and beans being the most toxic plant foods, and fruits generally being the least toxic types of plant foods (I'll explain more on that concept of plant toxicity levels in a bit)...

I've been intensely studying the science of carnivore and carnivore-ish (animal-based) diets for several years now, and have been fascinated by the impressive health benefits that thousands of people are getting from this way of eating. However, as with any way of eating, there are some types of people that get a lot more benefits than others.

The biggest categories of people that seem to benefit the most from animal-based diets are people with these conditions...

1. Autoimmune conditions -- a very high percentage of people with autoimmunity see a dramatic reduction in symptoms, and many times, and full resolution of symptoms by following either a carnivore diet or a mostly carnivore diet that contains only the simplest and least toxic plants. For autoimmunity, it's basically the most efficient type of elimination diet, since there's so many types of plants that trigger autoimmune symptoms.

It's fairly common for people with autoimmune conditions to get triggered by plant foods such as gluten-containing grains, beans (very high in lectins), nightshades (tomatoes, peppers, eggplant, and white potatoes), oxalates from leafy greens, and other problematic compounds in plants.

2. Gut/digestion issues -- since excessive fiber and excessive plant-based antinutrients and plant toxins can worsen digestive conditions, a mostly meat diet can actually be really healing for the digestive system in a lot of people, even though that statement surprises most people. Even the world-renowned digestive doctor Dr. Michael Ruscio stated in an interview that somewhere around 60% or more of his patients need less fiber, not more. Too much fiber can cause overgrowths of certain types of bacteria that can cause more digestive distress. Too much fiber can also irritate the digestive tract in a lot of people as well.

I personally know a LOT of people that are using carnivore diets and experiencing dramatically improved digestion. I also know several people with Crohn's disease where carnivores are the only thing that has worked for them to control their Crohn's, and they had tried everything before that.

It won't work for everyone, and most conventional doctors have never even heard of carnivore diets, so don't expect your doctor to know anything about it if you ask. In fact, most conventional doctors (I'd say 95% of them) don't know much at all about nutrition since there's almost zero nutrition education in medical school. So the only MDs that know a lot about nutrition are usually just the small percentage of them that are self taught.

3. Diabetes and obesity -- although carbs aren't "bad" necessarily, especially for metabolically healthy people or people that do intense exercise, low-carb diets (including carnivore type low-carb diets) can be particularly powerful for at least some time frame for getting type 2 diabetics back to normal blood sugar and insulin functioning in the body. If you're diabetic or pre-diabetic, I'd highly recommend reading this natural method for reversing Diabetes here.

Also, weight loss gets pretty darn easy when you're eating almost entirely meat, because meat is the single most satiating food you can eat, and it's basically impossible to overeat on calories with a meat-only or mostly meat diet. Think about how hard it is to overeat on steak. You just simply stop when you're full. But think how easy it is to overeat on mac n cheese, cereal, bagels, bread, pizza, ice cream, and other carb/fat combos that are highly addicting. I know personally when I have pizza, bread, or pasta in front of me, I can't stop eating it because it's so addictive, and I end up over-stuffing myself with thousands of excess calories. But with a juicy grass-fed steak, I just eat until I'm satisfied and then naturally stop.

As for me personally, I've done about an 85-90% carnivore diet for about 3 years now (I'd call it animal-based, with only carefully selected plants such as fruit that I know does well with my body)... For me, this has been the absolute easiest and best diet for me, and I've never felt so good. My digestion is basically almost perfect since cutting out most veggies, beans, nightshades, etc, and my energy and body composition have improved as well. And my bloodwork has been nearly perfect too for these last few years on a mostly meat-based diet.

And no, despite the false belief by outdated doctors and the mainstream media that cholesterol causes heart disease, nothing could be further from the truth... in fact, the biggest causes of heart disease are actually plant foods like vegetable oils and sugar, but NOT meat. Meat, fish, and eggs actually contain important nutrients that can help prevent heart disease, such as vitamin K2, carnosine, carnitine, DHA/EPA, stearic acid, etc.

As for what I personally eat... I eat mostly red meat almost every day (grass fed beef, bison, lamb, and yak), fish and shellfish a couple times a week, eggs, and the only plants I eat are small amounts of squash, sweet potatoes, carrots, avocado, cucumbers, coffee, wine, and sweet fruit only during the local fruit season, but not during winter. I also enjoy a small spoonful of honey a few days a week as a dessert replacement.

I personally choose to avoid chicken and pork mostly, since they have about 10x the inflammatory omega6 content of red meat (red meat only contains 2-3% omega6, whole chicken and pork contain about 15-20%, since chicken and pork are fed almost entirely grains and soy, whereas red meat like beef, lamb and bison eats mostly grass and forage for the majority of their lives)... I explain in more detail why RED meat is healthier than chicken or pork in this article, and also why red meat is more environmentally sustainable too, which surprises most people.

The best diet change I ever made that had the biggest impact on improving my health was cutting out most veggies and beans over the last 3-4 years. I actually intentionally avoid almost all veggies and beans now, and this had the most dramatic improvement on how I've felt on a daily basis.

I personally don't think veggies are an ancestrally consistent food source for humans, and a study of over 300 hunter-gatherer tribes showed that the average diets of hunter-gatherers around the world was about 80-85% meat, fish, and fruit, and the other 15% was basically small amounts of nuts and roots... But hunter gatherers really didn't eat much of what we'd call "vegetables" in our modern day food supply. Leaves and stems were only 1% of the average hunter-gatherer diet, even in tropical areas.

After all, 99% of leaves in the wild are toxic, and why would hunter-gatherers have wasted time and energy gathering something that has no calories...it just makes no logical sense. The majority of plant foods our ancestors ate was actually fruit mostly (the only part of the plant that wants to be eaten so we can spread the trees seed elsewhere), along with a little bit of nuts and roots, since those are the more calorically-dense plants that would have made sense to gather.

I also think that about 50% of vegetables are actually harmful to a lot of people based on genetics and other health conditions... For example, brassica veggies can be bad for people with thyroid conditions, nightshade veggies can be bad for people with arthritis, leafy greens can cause oxalate issues such as kidney stones, and certain other vegetables can often worsen digestive issues. So as you can see, veggies can often have more detrimental effects than benefits.

Another thing I have noticed over the years is that the majority of men in general seem to do fantastic on carnivore or mostly carnivore diets, whereas women seem to be more 50/50... Some women feel amazing about carnivores, and other women feel the need for more fiber and more plant foods in general. This is actually ancestrally consistent too, since hunter-gatherers generally had the men as the main hunters and the women more frequently as gatherers, and the men had access to more frequent meat than the women in a lot of these tribes. So it's possible that men are built for a slightly higher protein diet than women as a generalization.

Another good example is my friend Dr Paul Saladino, who wrote the popular book The Carnivore Code... he's been mostly carnivore for 3 years now too, and eats nothing but meat, organs, honey, and a small amount of fruit, and the guy is one of the healthiest people I know, whereas when he was vegan I think 6 or 7 years ago, he destroyed his health eating that way.

Lastly, I'd recommend people have an open mind when researching things like carnivore vs plant-based diets, as there's a LOT of closed-mindedness from the plant-based community to even consider or research anything other than what the biased information they currently believe. I've come to the conclusion that most humans can thrive just fine on either a meat-based diet or possibly even a plant-based diet as long as those plants are considered on a scale of plant toxicity and chosen carefully, while also getting at least some animal-based foods to balance out the micronutrients that simply can't be obtained from plants only. And some people (if you have northern genetics) might even consider being more animal-based in the winter and early spring, when our northern european ancestors would have been mostly carnivore, and then switching to a higher plant diet in the summer and fall when fruits, nuts and roots would have been more plentiful.

Another thing is that it seems more important for longevity that we're careful about avoiding the WORST foods that are causing most disease... with the absolute worst foods that are killing most people being vegetable oils (aka seed oils like soybean oil, corn oil, sunflower oil, cottonseed, canola, etc) and sugar, and possibly too much refined grains too. And for people that try out eating a more meat-based diet (with smaller amounts of carefully selected plant foods), they often find that it becomes really easy to avoid the worst foods like vegetable oils and sugar because they don't need to eat any processed food and also don't have cravings for unhealthy food anymore either since meat is so satiating.

<u>5 Liver-Damaging Foods you MUST AVOID</u>

Your liver works hard for you your whole life, but what have you done for your liver?

An oft-overlooked organ, The Centers for Disease Control recently named your liver "one of the largest and most important organs…"

Which makes sense…considering it does a multitude of essential tasks that keep your body running smoothly:

Regulates hormone levels
Helps rid the body of waste or "toxins"
Builds proteins and makes bile, which helps you absorb fats
Adjusts cholesterol levels
Stores sugar for when you really need it
Filters and removes bacteria from your blood…

For your liver, all of this and more is simply in a day's work...

Unfortunately, the American Liver Foundation recently shared these scary stats at the end of 2021:

100 million+ Americans have a fatty liver
20 million+ will develop liver fibrosis disease as a result

5 million+ will progress to cirrhosis and possible end-stage liver failure Some will be lucky enough to be listed for transplant, which is the only cure, but ~30% of those who do will die waiting

The good news is, if you want to do your liver a favor and take important steps to avoid a lifetime of weight gain & health problems…

<u>"What you eat can have a profound impact on how effective (or ineffective) your liver is," says Dr. Walding:</u>

For this reason, being aware of the foods that slow your liver processing can help you make healthy decisions about your diet…

And ultimately make your liver (and you) much "happier."

To guide you in this effort, we recommend you to print this list of the most liver-damaging foods to avoid…

First, Here's a Look at 5 Surprising Dietary Culprits That Can Do Irreversible Damage to Your Liver.

1.) Crackers: This popular snack may seem innocent enough, but they're not an excellent option for your liver health. Any foods with refined carbs or sugars, can be problematic for the liver, according to research. It can be easy to just munch on crackers mindlessly, but keep your hard-working liver in mind the next time you reach for a sleeve.

2.) Salted or Cured Meats: Too much fatty meat and/or salt is a problem for the liver, says The American Liver Foundation*, so it should go without saying that cured meats like prosciutto, or even cold cuts like ham, bologna, or salami, are all foods that are best eaten sparingly. Instead, opt for high-quality, lean meats like chicken, turkey, or seafood.

3.) Fruit Cups
This one may come as a surprise. According to a 2013 study*Over-consumption of fruits can actually introduce too much fructose to the body, which the liver may have issues processing and can result in fatty liver

issues. Canned and packaged fruits are also often packed with artificial sweeteners and added sugars.

4.) Common Condiments
It's not just the obvious sources of sugar in your diet that could be causing serious damage to your liver. Often the more dangerous sources of fructose are those in which the sugar content is less obvious, such as ketchup & salad dressings. Just one tablespoon of Heinz Ketchup contains 4 grams of sugar, and one serving of Kraft Creamy French Salad Dressing, for example, delivers 6 grams of sugar.

5.) Vegetable and Seed Oils
Sunflower, corn, soybean, and "vegetable" oils are omega-6 polyunsaturated fatty acid (PUFA)-rich. The American Society for Nutrition found in 2020* that this, "...fatty acid composition rather than the amount of fat, may actually be the key factor inducing obesity." Widespread overuse of these oils has also been implicated in the rise of system-wide inflammation, modern lifestyle diseases, and contributing to liver damage by way of non-alcoholic fatty liver disease. Even worse, when heated, the polyunsaturated omega-6 fats found in these common cooking oils generate a substance known as hydroxynonenal, which researchers now believe plays a key role in cell degeneration and cell death*.

What You Can Do to Naturally Boost & Protect the Health of Your Liver

Due to a severe incline in environmental toxins, sedentary lifestyles, and the prevalence of obesity, diabetes, and metabolic syndrome…

The annual increase in the incidence of Non-Alcoholic Fatty Liver Disease (NAFLD) has become a global public health problem.

As the name implies, the main characteristic of NAFLD is too much fat stored in your liver cells…

In extreme cases, this alone results in abdominal pain, nausea, yellowish skin and whites of the eyes (jaundice), swollen abdomen and legs (edema), extreme tiredness or mental confusion, and weakness…

But more often progresses into dangerous liver inflammation, advanced scarring (cirrhosis), and liver failure.

A fatty liver is also associated with high levels of fat in your bloodstream (triglycerides)…

Which is a huge concern as medical experts call high triglycerides "a 'silent' problem with big implications" such as a four-fold increase in the likelihood of having a heart attack or stroke.

Not only that, high levels of extra flabby fat stored throughout your body is known to raise your blood sugar levels, which can lead to pre-diabetes and, eventually, type 2 diabetes…

Plus cause inflammation of the pancreas (a condition which doctors call pancreatitis) and permanent tissue damage.

Currently, there is no registered drug for the treatment of NAFLD, so it is essential for Americans to tailor their diets to safeguard the health of their liver.

"Frozen" Nutrient to Help Prevent Liver Fat Buildup

Fatty fish is ironically great for lowering the levels of fat in your liver…

And if you're as health-conscious as I think you are--you probably already know it's because of the high levels of omega-3 essential fatty acids that fish contains.

In a review of ten randomized controlled trials, omega-3 fatty acid supplementation was shown to:

Reduce inflammation
Enhance insulin sensitivity
Lower blood triglyceride levels*…

These are 3 KEY factors to naturally improve & protect the health of your liver.

Unfortunately, only certain types of fatty or oily fish contain enough of the right types of omega-3s to make a difference in your liver health…

And many ALSO contain contaminants like mercury, dioxins, and pesticides.

Considering these issues, it is not so shocking that even with all we know about the POWER of omega-3s… 80% of Americans still do not have enough of them in their diet.

Fortunately, breakthrough research has revealed a secret "frozen" source way out in the

Antarctic Ocean that science has shown to contain THE MOST POWERFUL omega-3s found in nature…

And incorporating it into your nightly routine has been proven to help you avoid the 3 top causes of NAFLD.

In fact, the meta-analysis mentioned above proved that the two types of omega-3s found in this Antarctic supernutrient even significantly decreased the amount of liver fat observed on ultrasound.

So, What is the Best Form of Omega-3s to Support Liver Health? Here's a hint:

It's not fish oil.

The purest most effective form of omega-3s come from a unique oceanic organism that is found only in the pristine frozen waters of the antarctic ocean:

Wild-caught krill.

Otherwise known as the #1 "frozen" supernutrient for abundant liver health.

Krill oil contains high levels of the omega-3 fatty acids EPA and DHA which have been shown to help support healthy liver function.

Because krill are sourced from the Antarctic ocean, they're virtually free of toxins – making them far more pure and potent than other omega-3 sources like fish oil.

Research suggests that the fatty acids found in wild-caught krill can help reduce inflammation, improve liver enzyme levels and help protect against certain liver diseases.

Even better…

Krill oil also contains a special antioxidant that fish oil lacks…

It's called astaxanthin – a powerful antioxidant that can help protect liver cells from oxidative damage.

The Astaxanthin Found Only In Krill Oil Has Been Shown To Support Liver Health In Several Ways...

First, it has strong antioxidant properties, which can help protect the liver from oxidative damage caused by free radicals.

It also has anti-inflammatory properties, which can help reduce inflammation of the liver.

Additionally, astaxanthin has been shown to reduce levels of fat accumulation in the liver, which can help improve overall liver function.

Common Causes of Bad Breath (and How to Freshen Up)

According to science, bad breath, or halitosis, occurs at the microbial level. Bad breath is a result of the bacteria in our mouths breaking down lingering food particles in between our teeth, on our gums and tongue.

When this happens, sulfuric compounds are released, giving off a bad odor and producing what we know as bad breath, or what medical practitioners refer to as halitosis.

From a more holistic perspective, looking to the wisdom of Ayurveda (Ancient Indian Medicine) they would also agree with these statements. Practitioners of Ayurveda suspect that poor oral hygiene and surprisingly enough, poor digestive function, are the primary causes of bad breath.

Let's explore these causes a bit more, along with 12 others. We will also look at some holistic solutions for overcoming bad breath.

14 Reasons You Might Have Bad Breath

1. You Just Woke Up:
This is perhaps the most obvious cause right here. But let's take a look at why this is: during sleep, the body is actually busy at work detoxifying, repairing, and regenerating tissues.

The bacteria in the mouth are quite awake, as well. This is due to the fact that saliva production dramatically slows during sleep. Because saliva has a major role in cleaning the mouth and keeping pathogens from thriving, there can be a buildup of bacteria after sleeping.

Solution
If this is the case, then have no fear, morning breath is completely normal for most people and can be reversed with simple morning oral hygiene practices like oil pulling.

2. Mouth-Breathing

Chronically breathing through the mouth may lead to dry mouth by inhibiting saliva production. Dry mouth, as we'll discuss, is a major cause of bad breath.

If the mouth is overly dry from mouth breathing, then it loses its ability to properly eliminate leftover food particles.

One German study actually showed that those who spent a lot of time in physical training were more likely to have cavities – which can be a cause of bad breath. The researchers considered that the heavy mouth breathing results in low saliva production.

Solution

While breathing may be simple, many people do it only automatically. Better to practice more conscious breathing, particularly during exercise. It's best to take deep breaths from the diaphragm through the nose to avoid dry mouth.

3. Stinky Foods

Sometimes bad breath is as simple as the foods we eat. Common stinky foods like garlic and onions are infamous for producing unwelcomed breath.

However, there are also other culprits, including certain spices and cruciferous veggies like cabbage, cauliflower, and Brussels sprouts. These foods are also high in sulfur, which can produce an unpleasant odor.

As we will discuss later, bad breath can stem from the digestive tract, so while these foods may not be unpleasant to taste, burping them up later can produce an off-putting sulfur smell. When you eat these particular foods, the sulfuric compounds are absorbed into the bloodstream then into the lungs, where they can be expelled even hours after consuming them.

Solution
Chew sugar-free gum after a particularly stinky meal. This stimulates the production of saliva to prevent foul mouth odors.

4. Smoking

Time to add to the list of health conditions that can be caused by cigarettes.
Unsurprisingly, smoking not only increases the amount of odor-producing
compounds in a person's mouth and lungs, but the habit can also dry out
your mouth, leading to lower saliva production, according to a 2004 review
by researchers from Hong Kong.

Solution
There are more serious reasons to quit smoking than bad breath. We're not
going to run down the laundry list of why it's bad for your health but here
is a good place to start if you're trying to quit.

5. Medication

Certain meds—like some antihistamines, diuretics, antipsychotics, and
muscle relaxants—can cause side effects that include dry mouth, says Dr.
Rifai. And that, in turn, can reduce the amount of saliva your mouth
produces and increase the bacteria camping out there.

Solution
Since you can't do anything about your medication regimen, try cleaning
your tongue with either a toothbrush or a tongue scraper. According to the
American Dental Association, your tongue harbors most of the bacteria
that causes smelly breath, and scraping it off the surface may halt bad
breath, at least temporarily.

6. Sinus Infection/Cold

The mucus in your nose helps filter all the foreign particles that you
breathe in from the environment—a good thing. But what happens when
that mucus starts building up in the back of your throat because you have
terrible pollen allergies or a nasty cold?

Those foreign particles eventually travel into your mouth, settle on the
surface of your tongue, and in turn trigger bad breath, according to one

2012 review in the International Journal of Oral Science. As if a sore throat wasn't bad enough.

Solution
Use a saline nasal wash to help clear your nasal passages but if the problem persists, see your doctor.

7. A Low-Carb Diet

People who slash their carbohydrate intake have been known to report increased levels of halitosis. And, in fact, when researchers from Yeshiva University compared subjects on a very low-carb diet to those on a low-fat diet, they found that more people in the former group reported having bad breath than the latter.

However, it should also be noted that the low-fat dieters also confessed to more burping (and, um, farting.)

Solution
If a low-carb diet is working for you, sugar-free gum and drinking more water will help mask the order.

8. Cavities

Your mom has already warned you that a buildup of plaque can erode your teeth, leaving you with cavities. And while poor oral hygiene certainly contributes to bad breath, those "holes" may also trigger halitosis indirectly, too: "Food can get caught in the cavities," explains Dr. Grbic, and since cavities can be hard to clean, the remnants of your last meal can linger there for longer-than-usual periods of time, which can then lead to more bad breath. (For the record, yes, you'll need a filling.)

Solution
For fresh breath, following proper oral hygiene habits is very important. Proper brushing, flossing, and tongue scraping are a few ways to prevent odor-inducing bacteria from building up on the teeth and tongue.

9. Dental Appliances

We're not just talking about braces—orthodontic appliances like dentures and fixed bridges can be difficult to maintain, too. (Research also shows that dental appliances are linked with higher amounts of plaque accumulation—which is why a good cleaning regimen is so important.)

Solution
It's important that you clean them every day, says Dr. Grbic, as they're also prime magnets for food particles, which can become lodged in the material.

10. Alcohol

Alcohol lingers on your breath long past last call. In fact, one 2007 study by researchers from Israel found that drinking alcohol was linked to increased rates of halitosis—this despite the fact that their subjects had fasted for 12 hours overnight and were also allowed to brush their teeth in the morning.

The study authors suspected that not only does booze dry out a person's mouth, but that a certain odor is triggered when the body metabolizes alcohol.

Solution
If you tend to get unusually smelly breath after drinking, stick to a limit and don't go past it. Also, a glass of water between drinks not only helps keep bad breath at bay, but also helps control your alcohol intake by making you more full.

11. Heartburn or Acid Reflux

The overwhelming majority of halitosis cases are caused by the bacteria in a person's mouth—but researchers also suspect that in a minority of people, bad breath is triggered by a GI disorder like gastroesophageal reflux disease (GERD), in which the contents of a person's stomach leak back up into the esophagus.

One 2007 study published in the journal Oral Diseases found that bad breath was more prevalent in people with GERD than those with other digestion problems, possibly because the disease may damage a person's throat tissue.

Solution
Avoid foods that may aggravate acid reflux. This includes spicy foods, alcohol, fruit juices, and coffee. [tweet_quote] Eating foods that are rich in fiber also helps your digestion run well and prevent reflux. [/tweet_quote] Instead of reaching for an overly sugary drink, drinking (still, not carbonated) water will be easier on your stomach and also help wash away stinky bacteria.

12. Strep Throat

Strep is a bacterial infection, not a viral one, and those invading bugs can cause your breath to smell bad, says Dr. Grbic. Not only that, but other kinds of sinus infections can turn into bacterial ones that produce a smelly, pus-like type of mucus. (Sorry for the visual.)

Plus, some of these infections are also associated with specific types of bacteria that are known to produce a particularly bad odor in a person's mouth.

Solution
To wash away bacteria lingering in your mouth, brush your teeth daily, scraping your tongue each time, and to gargle with water after each meal.

13. Poor Digestive Health

A healthy digestive system is crucial for optimal overall health. In your gut there are trillions of beneficial bacteria that influence many of your body functions, including your immune system.

Studies show that an estimated 80 percent of your immune system is located in your gut. The ratio of good and bad gut bacteria is a crucial indicator of the condition of your health.

Your gut should have a balance of somewhere near 85 percent good
bacteria and 15 percent bad. An imbalance between good and bad bacteria
can predispose you to a wide number of health problems more serious than
bad breath and body odor.

Having less-than-optimal gut flora can make you vulnerable to health
conditions linked to bad breath. A fishy smell in the breath suggests kidney
problems, while fruity-smelling breath may mean uncontrolled diabetes.

Solution
This is why reseeding your gut with beneficial bacteria is essential for
optimal health and disease prevention. But before I enumerate the steps
that will help you achieve this, you must first understand how your diet
plays a significant role in the imbalance of your gut flora.

14. Compromised Immunity

At the core of overall good health is a well-functioning immune system.
Essentially, our immune system keeps building antibodies to protect the
body from being taken over by pathogens.

Many autoimmune disorders and any time of weakened immunity are
connected to halitosis. This is on the basis that bad bacteria in the mouth
are not being handled properly by the immune system.

Solution
To say the least, there is a strong correlation between the immune system
and dental health. If you suspect this is the case, then stick to building your
immunity up with gentle exercise, good sleep, and other basic healthy
lifestyle habits.

Seven More Reasons to Love Avocados That You Didn't Already Know

Avocados have become the darling of the many healthy and weight loss diets, as well as being a staple of the Paleo diet. They are having their 'moment' in the spotlight for sure! And for good reason! We all know that they are very healthy for us, low glycemic/low carb and full of super nutrients like healthy monounsaturated fats, vitamins, minerals, antioxidants and serious phytochemicals, but wait—there's more!

Avocados have been gaining steadily in popularity over the last ten years. In fact, the rate of consumption of avocados has about doubled in the last ten years and demand keeps growing! Mexico and Latin America are some of the biggest suppliers along with California. Did you know that there are actually over a thousand different types of avocados, but here in the United States, we mainly see the popular Hass avocado most of the time. Although the demand has gone up for this buttery fruit, supplies this year are lower, so you may be paying a higher price for your avo—but they are well worth it for your health and your body!

Here's a few reasons why:

1. Avocados Stabilize Blood Sugar and

Fight Metabolic Syndrome
The healthy fats and other nutrition you get from avocados help your body to stabilize blood sugar and insulin, helping fight diabetes and metabolic syndrome, as well as contributing to fat loss and muscle building. They are low glycemic; therefore no rise in blood sugar and no fat-storing insulin release. The healthy fat content in avocados makes you feel full longer and cuts down on food cravings, so that makes it a perfect food if you are trying to burn fat and lose weight—even though avocados are considered fairly calorically dense. All in all, researchers discovered that avocado consumers were 50 percent less likely to develop metabolic syndrome than people who don't normally eat them! The blood sugar stabilizing

effect avocados have also helps reduce blood pressure, LDL cholesterol, and triglycerides.

A study published in Nutrition Journal (January 2013), made up of 17,567 participants, also found that avocado-eaters generally eat a more balanced diet than non-avocado consumers, had significantly higher intakes of vegetables and fruit, and had higher intakes of vitamins, minerals and other antioxidants. BMI and body weight were significantly LESS in people who eat avocados on a regular basis. Speaking of high-fat foods that actually HELP you to get leaner, here are 7 fatty foods that fight aging and flatten your stomach (some will surprise you!)

2. Cancer Prevention

The Journal of Nutrition and Cancer recently published the results of a study, showing avocados as a major player in cancer-fighting and study results show phytochemicals as powerful as some chemotherapy! Other research suggests that phytochemicals extracted from avocados help induce cancer cell cycle death, inhibit growth, and induce apoptosis in precancerous and cancer cell lines.

Avocados' abundance of monounsaturated fats also help fight cancer by being an effective anti-inflammatory agent. Beta-sitosterol also protects the prostate gland in men, fighting cancer and improving immune functions. And the powerful carotenoids fight skin cancer, as well as aging.

3. Weight Loss—Really!!

While avocados get a bad rap because they are calorically dense and high in fats, they are actually a great weight loss food. Diets lower in carbohydrates have actually been shown to help in fat loss, and in reducing hunger because they keep blood sugar and fat-storing insulin in check. Fats are super filling and increase satisfaction that help you eat less overall. And they allow you to go longer between meals without getting hungry. That healthy fat also helps your body absorb more fat-burning vitamins and minerals as well.

A study conducted in 2005, examined the effects of avocados, a rich source of calories coming from monounsaturated fatty acids, as part of an energy-restricted diet on weight loss, serum lipids and vascular function in overweight and obese subjects. They found that consumption of 30 grams a day of fat from avocado within a restricted calorie diet didn't compromise weight loss at all when substituted for 30 grams a day of mixed dietary fats. The diet high in avocado resulted in significant weight loss in addition to other health improvements. Measurements including body mass, body mass index and percentage of body fat decreased significantly in both groups during the study. Only the avocado test group experienced positive changes in fatty acid blood serum levels. So, there are clearly avocado benefits for weight loss!

4. Avocados Contain Amazing Facts

Avocados contain oodles of oleic acid, the same type of healthy fat that is in olive oil, which helps—among other things—lower bad cholesterol and fight cancers. Unlike saturated fats or highly processed vegetable oils, avocado oil regulates blood sugar, protects the heart as well as the brain. Avocados contain plenty of oleic acid, the same monounsaturated fat in olive oil, that helps lower cholesterol and is helpful in preventing breast cancer and other cancers.

Avo's help to block the development of arteriosclerosis (the gunk inside your blood vessels that blocks blood flow) partly because of their blood sugar-lowering effects. Other serious health-protecting ingredients include fiber, beta-sitosterol, magnesium, and potassium, which help to regulate blood pressure and lower LDL cholesterol. This study shows people eating avocados dropped total cholesterol by 17%, LDL's decreased by 22%, triglycerides by 22%, and healthy HDL rose by 11%. That avo fat is GOOD for you!!

5. Healthy Babies—Before and After Birth

One medium avocado has about a quarter of your required daily amount of folate, or folic acid, a B vitamin that plays an essential role in making new cells by helping to produce healthy DNA and RNA. Folate is required for pregnant women, and helps lower the risk of birth defects in babies, as well as being important for heart health.

And avocados are the perfect baby food as well! They are firm enough to be picked up by tiny fingers, but easily mashable and edible—even for someone with no teeth! What's more, we now know they are chock full of healthy nutrition, healthy fats and massive phytochemicals. And their mild taste is something babies love, making avo's a great baby superfood!

6. Eye Health
Avocados have lots of carotenoids and lutein, antioxidants that are both valuable for healthy eyes. It also contains zeaxanthin, alpha-carotene and beta-carotene, plus significant quantities of vitamin E. The oleic acid in avo's helps the body absorb those precious carotenoids and convert to vitamin A, as well as being able to access the antioxidants in other foods as well. Carotenoid benefits include lowering inflammation, promoting healthy growth and development, and boosting immunity, among others.

7. Healthy Inside and Healthy

Outside—Skin and Hair
Avocados' load of phytochemicals and antioxidants fight damage from the sun and the environment by reducing inflammation and DNA damage. People who eat diets rich in antioxidants as well as healthy fats have healthier, less wrinkly skin than people who eat the Standard American Diet (SAD). In addition, the healthy carotenoids in colorful veggies, including avocados add a rich, healthy golden glow to your skin. And, because of the rich oils and vitamins in avocados, you can mash one up and use it as a moisturizing, calming facial mask as well!

Avocados' massive supply of phytonutrients including their polyphenols and flavonoids also help fight osteoarthritis, and other inflammatory degenerative diseases.

Avocados' growing popularity has created a serious worldwide craving for this buttery orb, so countries like Mexico and many other South American countries have been gearing up their production. However, avocados—especially American Hass avocados use more water than the South

American varieties, so California avocados may be in short supply this year. Rising demand and avocado prices are actually fueling illegal deforestation in some parts of the world, and drug and mafia cartels are at work to control the supply of this popular food. High demand and lowered supply may mean your favorite avo prices could rise. Careful handling, a watchful eye that they don't get overripe and knowing how to store your leftover avocado will help to prevent wasting these lovelies.

What About That Pit?
A study by Pennsylvania State University revealed that avocado pits, or seeds, have been used medicinally for generations. Avocado pits in South America have been used as a treatment for inflammation, diabetes and hypertension. This mostly unused element of the fruit contains phenolic compounds, which are known to prevent cancer, cardiovascular disease and other degenerative illnesses. But beware, some food experts warn against eating the pits thinking that it may cause intestinal discomfort or other health issues. More research is needed at this point on the detriments or benefits of eating the seeds of avocados.

We all want to stay young and healthy forever. But unfortunately, that isn't entirely possible. Longevity is a hot topic these days, and there are many lifestyle habits, dietary habits, and natural and pharmaceutically based supplements and treatments on the horizon that can be used as powerful tools to slow down the aging process.

The anti-aging industry is a hugely popular growing industry. Successful aging is one of the most important areas of health with our fast-aging population. There are currently 671 million people who are over the age of 60, worldwide.

What is Longevity?
While we all would like to live long, productive lives, many struggle just managing chronic disease that seems to arrive with aging. Longevity is not just about living as long as possible, but living the longest, healthiest life possible—free of chronic diseases.

This is where the term "health span" comes in. Many may agree that a person's health span is far more important than the life span. However, being "healthy" means different things to different people. A better definition of longevity might include being free from serious disease, having energy and cognitive processes, as well as physical mobility and strength.

Successful aging means having a healthy physical body and good mental health. What's interesting however, is that when we do things that are healthy for our physical bodies, these actions benefit our brain health as well. And vice versa.

We die not of old age, but of the cumulative failures within our cells. These failures are not inevitable breakdowns, but instead are the reversible elements of aging.

Lifestyle habits accumulate, and those habits can either have a negative effect on health or a positive one. Small daily habits can be cumulative and build up to big things over a lifetime. The best habits to include in your day-to-day life right now are, regular exercise, maintaining your steady blood sugar and a healthy diet, regular social contact, and good sleep on a regular basis.

Building on top of this foundational healthy habits are some ground-breaking scientific treatments worth mentioning that all point towards increased health and longevity.

1. Exercise

Exercise, for example, is one of the best ways to help protect both our physical health AND our mental health. While you probably already know that exercise can contribute to a longer healthier life, more and more research points to how and why exercise is so beneficial.

Research from Harvard Medical School indicates that regular physical activity is linked to a longer lifespan. According to the study, people who exercise regularly for at least 30 minutes a day have a 20% lower risk of death than sedentary folks.

Another study from the Mayo Clinic finds similar results, showing that people who exercise regularly had a 25% lower risk of dying early compared to those who were inactive.

Ok, so what types of exercise affect longevity? Turns out, basically all kinds—although some forms of exercise are more beneficial than others.

Research shows that aerobic exercise, especially including interval training, such as HIIT (high intensity interval training), along with running and cycling, have serious longevity benefits. Aerobic exercise not only strengthens the heart and lungs but also reduces blood pressure, and increases circulation.

Strength training—or resistance training as it is often called, is associated with stronger muscles, better balance, stronger bones, and better mobility. Muscle mass and strength will naturally decline with aging, and it accelerates after the age of 60, if we don't try to counteract that. These changes can have dramatically negative effects on our health.

If we do not prioritize muscle strength maintaining muscle mass as we age, the risks of muscle loss multiply and are harder to overcome as we age. With loss of muscle, we lose balance, and eventually we lose mobility.

Muscle mass correlates with a decrease in all-cause mortality. In other words, the more muscle mass you have, the lower your risk of dying from any chronic disease than some of your peers. It only takes an hour of resistance exercise each week to decrease your mortality risk, but the ideal 75-150 minutes a week is even better. That's working out 3-5 times a week for only a half an hour.

One of the most significant benefits of exercise is that it promotes neurogenesis, which is the birth of new brain cells. This is astounding new research. If you want to prevent cognitive decline, exercise is an essential element to improving cognitive function.

Researchers have shown in animal studies that exercise actually increases the creation of new brain cells in the hippocampus, which is a small seahorse-shaped part of the brain that forms memories and storage.

Exercise also can improve the health and function of the synapses between neurons in this region, allowing you to think more quickly and more clearly as the brain cells communicate better.

Regular exercise, according to longitudinal studies in humans, can increase the size of the hippocampus and prefrontal cortex, both of which are susceptible to cognitive decline such as dementia and Alzheimer's disease.

Regular exercise helps your body and your brain to stay younger and the results can be dramatic.

2. Diet

Diet is the second most controllable factor in aging and longevity. Diet is key to a healthier and longer lifespan. Mounds of research point to the fact that diet has everything to do with whether you end up with a chronic disease or not—especially diseases like diabetes, heart disease, obesity, and cancer. Even contributing inflammatory diseases such as arthritis, autoimmune disease, dementia, and more are all controllable by diet–wholly or partially.

The most recent research looks at blood sugar, metabolism, and AMPK pathways. AMPK is adenosine monophosphate-activated protein kinase, otherwise known as "AMPK".

AMPK is found in every living cell of your body. And if you want to avoid the primary symptoms of aging, you will need to maintain optimal AMPK activity. How do we do that?

AMPK controls a wide variety of metabolic pathways that help us metabolize and utilize energy from food and how we store that energy. AMPK manages our cell's energy in order for it to function efficiently.

When activated, AMPK in turn releases additional energy from sources (fats and sugars) in our bodies. So activated AMPK helps keep us lean, energetic, and active while renewing our cells. AMPK activity declines rapidly with aging, and when excess calories are available, the end result is accelerated aging.

You CAN boost AMPK activity through exercise, fasting or overall calorie restriction. There are also supplements that boost AMPK activity as well, such as Berberine. Boosting AMPK helps to keep your cells younger to slow down aging.

The problem is that our sedentary lifestyles and overabundance of calories ages us much faster. High caloric intake drastically decreases AMPK. This is like eating yourself to death. Growing masses of fat in our bodies reduce insulin sensitivity and increase system wide inflammation, leading to the chronic diseases that come with aging, such as heart disease, diabetes, and cancer.

Blood sugar levels also affect the brain and are implicated as being a major player in Alzheimer's and other types of dementia and neurodegeneration, according to this study.

Research recently published in the Journal, Neurology, have new data that suggests modest increases in blood sugar among people in their 50s, 60s and 70s can have negative effects on memory.

Researchers found that if a person's A1C measurement (A1C is a common blood test that shows an average blood sugar level over a -three month period) goes from 5 percent, which is in the normal range, to just 5.6 percent, it was associated with worsening memory recall.

Increases in blood sugar or chronically elevated blood sugar also leads to increased inflammation, which as mentioned before, increases one's susceptibility to chronic disease and autoimmune disease.

Bottom line, keep blood sugar in the low end of a healthy range with diet, exercise, and intermittent fasting.

One other thing worth mentioning is the influx of 'Continuous Glucose Monitors' on the market. These are tiny devices that attach to the skin of the arm or abdomen. A small sensor inside monitors glucose, and an app in your phone can read glucose measurements. It also tracks glucose patterns over the course of a 24-hour period.

While these are available only through a prescription in the U.S., they are excellent methods of monitoring blood sugar, and discovering which foods raise blood sugar. The day is soon coming when these monitors will be available to the general public and will be excellent to help people lose weight and increase longevity.

3. Peptide Therapy

Peptides are another area of cutting-edge anti-aging therapy. What are peptides? Peptides are short chains of amino acids which form a protein. Peptides work at the cellular level and can have a massive effect on aging, disease, and general health. Peptides have been shown to impact many health issues including arthritis, diabetes, autoimmune disease, inflammation, the healing process, and cellular DNA.

Peptides are being used as a form of treatment for many different types of health conditions. Some peptides can encourage production of growth hormone in the body, which can help reduce inflammation and autoimmune disease.

Other peptides can be effective in the treatment of obesity, as certain types can encourage the death of excess fat cells. Some peptides are used to decrease wrinkles and make skin look younger. Another type of peptide is known to encourage the production of melanin which can then decrease risk of skin cancer. Others are therapeutic for different types of sexual dysfunctions.

Longevity medicine offers peptide treatments such as human growth hormone compounds like CJC 1295 + Ipamorelin, MK-677 Ibutamoren, IGF-1 LR3 + CJC 1295 + Ipamorelin, Sermorelin, IGF-1 LR3, and Ipamorelin, among others.

These compounds have been found to be safe and effective for things like hair growth, recovering from injuries, increasing cognitive function, stimulating the libido, and improving athletic performance. Other people report peptides aid in sleep, reduce muscle and joint inflammation and increase mental clarity and energy.

Peptide therapy will certainly become one of the preferred longevity treatments as it becomes more and more available.

4. Sleep

Many people view sleep as a luxury and only catch up on it on weekends when their exhausted bodies can get the rest they truly need. However, sleep is an absolute necessity when it comes to health and longevity.

People often overlook the potential long-term health consequences of insufficient sleep, and the impact that health problems can have on a person's overall time and productivity.

Getting insufficient sleep is cumulative and over time, medical conditions such as obesity, diabetes, heart disease and other inflammatory diseases can develop. Several studies have linked insufficient sleep and weight gain. For example, one study found that people who slept less than six hours a night on a consistent basis were more likely to be overweight, while those who slept an average of seven to eight hours a night had lower body fat.

Other studies have shown that people who sleep five hours or less a night were more likely to develop type 2 diabetes. Insufficient sleep is often accompanied by blood sugar fluctuations and cravings for carbohydrates and sweets—possibly due to the rise in cortisol and increase in inflammation that occurs with those who do not get enough sleep.

Even modestly reduced sleep is associated with a much greater risk of heart disease and risk of death from heart disease.

Sleep also plays a big role in immune function and increases the levels of many inflammatory factors. People who are sleep deprived are much more likely to catch viruses like colds and the flu.

Both rapid eye movement (REM) and non-REM (NREM) sleep have crucial roles in our physical, behavioral, metabolic, and cognitive function. Poor sleep can also reduce life expectancy solely because it can raise the risk of accidents and injuries. An analysis of data from three separate studies suggests that sleeping five or fewer hours per night can raise one's mortality risk by as much as 15 percent.

Sleep quality is also tied into skin cell function, and reduced sleep can make the skin more vulnerable to environmental damage and more prone to visible signs of aging such as wrinkles and sagging skin. Our bodies produce hormones during sleep such as human growth hormones that contribute to our youthful appearance, energy, and strength. In fact, research has shown that just a single night of sleep deprivation can speed up cellular aging.

Sleep helps us store memories, and organize information in our brains, and helps with cognitive function like problem solving and attention to details.

Sleep also protects the overall health of the brain. During the night, the brain works to clear out toxins in the brain which can build up during the waking hours. This includes proteins that can damage brain tissue and impair healthy cognition.

5. Heat Therapy

Saunas, red light therapy and cold plunges have become a tool for increased longevity. Heating or cooling the body can have major health benefits that contribute to healthier aging.

Saunas have been around for many years, and the Scandinavians are still big users of saunas. Much of the research from heat saunas comes from the Scandinavians.

Many studies have been published showing that regular sauna use improves health and longevity. Health benefits from saunas include better insulin sensitivity, which helps lower blood sugar, faster recovery from injuries, release of growth hormone, and increased neurogenesis, which is the creation of new brain cells.

Sauna bathing has been found to induce profound physiological effects on the body that increases longevity. The high temperatures from a sauna cause the blood vessels to dilate which improves circulation, lowers blood pressure, and helps the body to remove toxins.

Sauna heat reduces inflammation which is a primary cause of aging and chronic disease. The heat of the sauna relaxes muscles and promotes relaxation, reducing stress levels, and cortisol. Chronic stress has been linked to higher levels of inflammation and increased aging.

6. Red Light Therapy

Red light therapy is emerging as another type of longevity therapy.

Red light therapy has been shown to have anti aging health benefits including reducing inflammation, increasing collagen in the skin, promoting wound healing, and improving skin conditions such as acne and psoriasis.

It has also been found to be effective in reducing pain and stiffness associated with conditions such as arthritis, as well as increasing muscle strength and endurance. Other studies have shown that red light therapy can help improve mood and cognitive function, and may be beneficial for treating conditions such as seasonal affective disorder (SAD) and depression.

Anti Aging effects of red light therapy include:

Increased Mitochondrial function: red light therapy has been found to increase the activity of mitochondria, the powerhouses of the cells, which are known to play a role in aging.
Sirtuins activation: Red light therapy has been found to activate the Sirtuins family of proteins, which are known to play a role in aging and longevity.
Increased NAD+ levels: red light therapy has been found to increase NAD+ levels, which is a molecule that is known to play a role in aging.
Increased Autophagy: Red light therapy has been found to increase autophagy, a process of cell self-cleaning, which is known to be beneficial for longevity.

7. Cold Plunge Therapy

Cold exposure and ice baths are 'the' thing right now to increase metabolism, cure your depression and reduce inflammation. From enhanced longevity to better moods and improved focus, to improved metabolism, cold water seems to be the new cure-all.

Cold therapy seems to have the greatest benefits to the central nervous system, the cardiovascular system, and the immune system, rather than just muscles.

Cold therapy fans believe benefits that include:

Boosting immune function

Improved circulation
Lowered heart rate
Deeper sleep
Better focus
Boosting energy levels
Lowered inflammation
Improve metabolic function
Reduced depression, improves mood
Increase in confidence
Like saunas, cold exposure is a way of shocking the body—in a good way. This shock stimulates the 'fight or flight' response, which causes an adaptive response because the stressor is brief, compared to long term stress which wears the body down, mentally, and physically.

Cold exposure is considered a hormetic stressor. A hormetic stressor is a type of natural stress that creates a positive response in the body. As your heart rate and respiration increase to help keep you warm, blood flow and oxygen increase throughout the body. Norepinephrine floods the brain, which boosts focus, attention, and mood, while reducing pain and inflammation. This also creates a nice endorphin rush.

8. Bioidentical Hormone Therapy Treatments

A foundational part of antiaging practice is hormone replacement. While bioidentical and conventional hormone therapy treatments have been around for a long time, there is greater attention and acceptance of hormone therapy treatments in terms of longevity. Aging skin, as decreases in muscle mass, decreasing levels of bone mineral density (BMD), loss of sexual desire and erectile dysfunction, slowed intellectual activity, and depressed mood have all been related to this decrease in hormone production with age.

Hormone therapy treatments have traditionally been used to correct sex hormone deficiencies in men and women. Women often begin hormone therapy during perimenopause or menopause to treat symptoms of declining hormones. These symptoms include insomnia, hot flashes, memory lapses, brain fog, depression, anxiety, loss of libido and more.

Women's hormone replacement generally consists of estrogen, progesterone, and sometimes testosterone.

Additionally, women who are postmenopausal and not on hormone therapy are at a much higher risk for heart disease, osteoporosis, and some forms of cancer, including colorectal cancer.

Many men receive testosterone replacement therapy to boost testosterone, often due to declining testosterone levels that go with aging. For men, testosterone deficiency can cause erectile dysfunction, loss of libido, loss of motivation and drive, reduced muscle mass, and lowered response to exercise, depression, insomnia, and lowered bone mass.

In both men and women, hormone replacement therapy—especially bioidentical hormone replacement therapy has been used not only to diminish symptoms of low hormones but also to prevent or slow the potential for chronic diseases of aging, including osteoporosis, cancer, heart disease, muscle loss/sarcopenia and even cognitive decline.

Both men and women on HRT report feeling younger, having less aches, and pains, sleeping more soundly at night, more interest in sex, smoother, less wrinkled skin, and improved response to exercise with increased lean body mass and loss of fat.

In addition to sex hormone replacement therapy, doctors are also including DHEA (Dehydroepiandrosterone) which is a master hormone from which sex hormones are made, and growth hormone for added longevity benefits.

9. Other Longevity Practices

IV therapy treatment centers have sprung up across the country. While many health fanatics are flocking to these centers to get intravenous vitamins and other nutrients, these centers have an appeal for those seeking to slow aging and fight disease as well.

IV treatments include vitamin, antioxidants and mineral infusions, glutathione (a powerful antioxidant), and Ultraviolet blood irradiation. UBI was regularly used during the 1940's and 1950's to treat medical conditions including pneumonia, tuberculosis, infections, and cancer, and is becoming popular again. Other therapies include phospholipid IV therapy which removes stored toxins from heavy metals in the body's fat cells.

10. Young blood plasma

Young blood plasma is a newer treatment for aging, in which young blood donors' blood is transfused in people wishing to slow aging. Young blood infusions cost upwards of $8-10,000 per liter, and have been shown in animal studies to slow aging. Young blood plasma is generally considered to come from donors who are 20 years old or younger.

Blood plasma does contain many proteins, enzymes and other nutrients that control aging, slow disease processes, and increase health and wellbeing. While human studies are still limited, and ongoing, one study done on Alzheimer's patients transfused with young plasma showed very promising results.

Conclusion

New treatments for longevity, slowing aging, and preventing diseases that go with aging are flooding the horizon. This article covers but a few of the more common anti aging procedures available to the general public today.

With the aging population here in the U.S. and in Europe, I am certain that we will be seeing many, many more innovative longevity practices—and many that are truly effective in slowing the aging process. Some of these may cost hundreds of thousands of dollars.

More importantly—and much less expensive–maintaining healthy lifestyle habits such as regular cardio and weight resistance exercise, getting 7-8 hours sleep each night, eating a diet high in antioxidants and high-quality proteins and fats, and maintaining close social contacts, are the foundational habits that will sustain one's life, longevity, and good health for a long, long time—without spending thousands and thousands of dollars.

Chapter 8 *living a healthy lifestyle*

Salt is a vital electrolyte for our bodies to function—without salt, we die.

However, salt is almost always at the top of the "foods to avoid" list. It seems the entire medical profession and along with most dietitians and nutritionists hate salt. Why is salt looked at as such a terrible thing for your health? As always, there's more to the story and today's guest-blog dives deep into the conspiracies about salt from the medical establishment, and why you actually need to have it daily.

However, salt is almost always at the top of the "foods to avoid" list. It seems the entire medical profession and along with most dietitians and nutritionists hate salt. Why is salt looked at as such a terrible thing for your health?

Salt vs Sodium

Salt is not pure sodium. Salt is a natural product that contains sodium. Table salt (like Morton salt) contains around 97% sodium. Other types of salt like sea salt and Himalayan pink salt contain less sodium, but do contain a few other minerals including magnesium, potassium and small amounts of calcium.

The Salt and Blood Pressure Connection

During the 1980s, researchers conducted a large global study that studies salt intake and blood pressure. What was discovered was that groups of people from undeveloped countries who didn't use salt also had low blood pressure.

One of these groups were the Yanomami of the Amazon rainforest. The Yanomami have very low sodium in their urine, which indicates very low sodium consumption—and they have very low blood pressure. Even the very elderly Yanomami possess low blood pressure.

However, when you look at another group of primitive people, the Kuna of Panama, you see a slightly different story. The Kuna also consume a low sodium diet and have low blood pressure, but when certain groups of the Kuna had access to more generous amounts of salt, blood pressure still remained low. In other words, there doesn't seem to be a direct relationship between salt intake and blood pressure. It's quite possibly diet and other lifestyle factors as well.

Another study, a meta-analysis of 6,250 patients found no direct link between salt intake, high blood pressure and increased risk of heart disease. Like many of our dietary recommendations, we need to take other things into consideration.

Two other meta-analyses (analysis of multiple studies) found that sodium restriction reduced blood pressure 5.39 mm Hg for systolic (top number) blood pressure and reduced diastolic blood pressure (lower number) 2.82 mm Hg for those who already had hypertension. Sodium restriction dropped blood pressure only 2.42 mm Hg and down 1.00 mm Hg, in those with normal readings. Not much really.

In addition, restricting sodium intake can also increase triglycerides and LDL cholesterol, as well as causing elevated stress hormones.

However, increasing potassium intake (naturally found in fruit and vegetables) was associated with over a 7-point drop in systolic blood pressure and a 2-point drop in diastolic blood pressure, but only for people with hypertension. The takeaway here is that increased potassium (which a healthy diet provides) is more beneficial to lowering blood pressure than a salt-restricted diet.

Our Bodies Need Salt to Survive

The human body can't live without some sodium. Salt is necessary for nerve transmission and to help contract and relax muscle fibers—including the muscles in the heart.

Some of the signs of salt deficiency include:

Dehydration—the body cannot hold onto water as well without salt
Muscle cramps

Higher risk of heart attack

Headaches

Weakness

Inability to withstand heat, especially when exercising

Cognitive decline in elderly

Irritability

When sodium levels are low in the body, chemical and hormonal messages signal the kidneys and even our sweat glands to hold onto water to conserve sodium.

Many studies point to the fact that sodium has many benefits in the body. It can actually help you conserve water, and make you feel less thirsty. Salt has several other health benefits too. Let's explore some of those good things about salt:

Exercise performance and heat tolerance

Back when I used to race my bike in the heat of a St. Louis summer (think high 90's temps + humidity in the 90% range), the heat used to really get to me. I remember a few races where I just got too hot to continue and dropped out. I was overheated and out of energy.

Once I learned about salt loading before racing or training in the heat, it was a game-changer. The heat no longer bothered me, and I had tons more energy. Suddenly instead of dropping out of races, I started winning them.

Studies show that sodium loading before exercising in the heat increases the body's fluid volume and reduces the physiological strain on your body from the training. Sodium loading helps you work out harder, longer and more effectively. And guess what? This method works for you whether it's hot out or not.

Salt and Electrolytes

Sodium from salt, is an important source of necessary electrolytes. Without sufficient electrolytes you can experience irregular heartbeat, muscle cramps, fatigue, nausea, and even seizures. Sodium is an electrolyte which is also vital to maintain the proper fluid balance in our bloodstream, inside and outside our cells.

Sea salt is an excellent source of electrolytes, which has been shown to prevent muscle cramping during exercise. Sea salt contains sodium, magnesium, potassium, and calcium, all of which you need for optimal health. These minerals must come from your diet because your body can't create them.

Manage Stress Better

When we are stressed, our bodies have more of the hormone, cortisol circulating. When cortisol levels are high, you feel more stressed. Salt has been shown to help your body clear cortisol from the blood. The faster your body gets rid of cortisol, the better you feel. Low sodium diets are often associated with higher stress hormone levels, as well as depression and anxiety.

An experiment published in 1995 showed, for example, that when rats are put in stressful situations, they preferred to drink salty water rather than unsalted water. In another study, when wild rabbits were stressed, their sodium intake shot up.

In another 2014 study involving about 10,000 Americans, researchers found a relationship between salt intake and depression: women on low-sodium diets tended to be more depressed than women with a regular salt intake. People may be self-medicating with salt and not even know it.

Chronic stress does seem to increase cravings for salty food—unfortunately it's usually salty processed foods like pizza, chips, or French fries. No wonder college kids are binging on this type of food. Could stress be the reason why an awful lot of Americans are munching on salty junk food?

You don't have to mow through a bag of potato chips if you are stressed and craving salt. Grab a handful of healthy nuts or beef jerky to snack on. You can also just add a couple more grinds of fresh Himalayan salt to your healthy dinner or sprinkle some sea salt on those fresh veggies you are munching on.

Salt and Sex
Salt has been found to accelerate sexual maturation in animal models, resulting in more offspring. Male rats also tend to have increased sperm counts when on a higher sodium diet.

This 1991 experiment, on men whose sodium intake was lowered to 2.4 grams a day, complained of erectile dysfunction more often than those who consumed three grams a day. The ED was even worse when combined with a diuretic (used for hypertension) and the low-sodium diet.

Growth

However, salt is almost always at the top of the "foods to avoid" list. It seems the entire medical profession and along with most dietitians and nutritionists hate salt. Why is salt looked at as such a terrible thing for your health?

Salt vs Sodium
Salt is not pure sodium. Salt is a natural product that contains sodium. Table salt (like Morton salt) contains around 97% sodium. Other types of salt like sea salt and Himalayan pink salt contain less sodium, but do contain a few other minerals including magnesium, potassium and small amounts of calcium.

The Salt and Blood Pressure Connection

During the 1980s, researchers conducted a large global study that studies salt intake and blood pressure. What was discovered was that groups of people from undeveloped countries who didn't use salt also had low blood pressure.

One of these groups was the Yanomami of the Amazon rainforest. The Yanomami have very low sodium in their urine, which indicates very low sodium consumption—and they have very low blood pressure. Even the very elderly Yanomami possess low blood pressure.

However, when you look at another group of primitive people, the Kuna of Panama, you see a slightly different story. The Kuna also consume a low sodium diet and have low blood pressure, but when certain groups of the Kuna had access to more generous amounts of salt, blood pressure still remained low. In other words, there doesn't seem to be a direct relationship between salt intake and blood pressure. It's quite possibly diet and other lifestyle factors as well.

Another study, a meta-analysis of 6,250 patients found no direct link between salt intake, high blood pressure and increased risk of heart disease. Like many of our dietary recommendations, we need to take other things into consideration.

Two other meta-analyses (analysis of multiple studies) found that sodium restriction reduced blood pressure 5.39 mm Hg for systolic (top number) blood pressure and reduced diastolic blood pressure (lower number) 2.82 mm Hg for those who already had hypertension. Sodium restriction dropped blood pressure only 2.42 mm Hg and down 1.00 mm Hg, in those with normal readings. Not much really.

In addition, restricting sodium intake can also increase triglycerides and LDL cholesterol, as well as causing elevated stress hormones.

However, increasing potassium intake (naturally found in fruit and vegetables) was associated with over a 7-point drop in systolic blood pressure and a 2-point drop in diastolic blood pressure, but only for people with hypertension. The takeaway here is that increased potassium (which a healthy diet provides) is more beneficial to lowering blood pressure than a salt-restricted diet.

Low Sodium and Diabetes
People with type 2 diabetes have worsening outcomes when they follow a low salt diet. A 2011 study showed people with Type 2 diabetes are more likely to die prematurely on a low-salt diet due to higher all-cause and

cardiovascular mortality. Another study from Harvard linked low-salt diets to an immediate onset of insulin resistance, a precursor to Type 2 Diabetes. Guidelines for salt restriction for people with type 2 diabetes may need to be reconsidered.

Aldosterone levels

Low sodium conditions can increase the hormone aldosterone. Aldosterone is an adrenal hormone that helps the body preserve sodium when it is perceived to be scarce.

High aldosterone levels are also associated with insulin resistance, and aldosterone-blocking medications are being explored as potential treatments for vascular disease and hypertension.

What Kind of Salt to Use?

Avoid using processed table salt as it is higher in sodium, often has fillers and anti-coagulants and has a harsh, bitter taste. Better choices are natural salt such as these:

Natural sea salt contains many more beneficial minerals such as magnesium and calcium and even iodine. Sea salt generally has a milder, smoother taste as well.
Pink Himalayan salt is rich in minerals, containing all 84 essential trace elements required by your body.
Celtic sea salt is an unrefined, unprocessed type of salt, sourced from clean coastal waters in France. Containing unprocessed and naturally forming minerals, this gray Sea Salt is harvested and dried and ready to use.
Salt makes food taste better. Ever eat a steak without salt? It's bland and boring. Or try a plate of steamed veggies without salt. It's just not all that good.

You can attempt to drop your salt intake to try to lower your blood pressure, but your body has ways of maintaining the levels it needs to function. And, food doesn't taste as good, your performance in the gym and in bed may suffer, and your cortisol and insulin may go up.

Better yet, sticking to a low-carb, primal, paleo style diet with few carbs, no grains or sugar will actually help your body clear out salt quicker and, in the process, you will get healthier, your blood pressure goes down and cardiovascular markers start looking up. Enjoy your salt with a healthy diet!

Chapter 9 *living a healthy lifestyle*

Alfred E. Newman had it right when he said,"We are living in a world today where lemonade is made from artificial flavors and furniture polish is made from real lemons." Too true. So when life gives you lemons, eat them whole and fresh!

All about lemons

The lemon was first created as a cross between a lime and a citron, and all three grow on evergreen shrubs. The Arabs introduced this small citrus fruit to the Europeans, who then brought them to Spain in the 11th century.

Along with other fruits and vegetables, Christopher Columbus brought lemons with him on his second voyage to the New World in 1493. They have been growing in Florida since the 16th century.

Besides large amounts of vitamin C, lemons contain riboflavin, thiamin, iron, magnesium, pantothenic acid, fiber, vitamin B6, potassium, copper, calcium and folate. Lemons even protected miners against scurvy during the California Gold Rush. They cost as much as one dollar each in 1849. Although we may not be overly concerned about scurvy in America today, here are 11 other great reasons why lemons should be a part of your healthy diet:

8 Ways to Treat Your Skin Right with Cucumbers

Cucumbers not only offer lots of nutrition for the body, they are known to be extremely beneficial to the skin.

Cucumber flesh contains vitamin C and caffeic acid which are known to help soothe skin irritations and reduce swelling in addition to preventing water retention. Cucumbers are also known to have nourishing, hydrating and astringent properties.

Consider one or more of these eight great ways to treat your skin right with this beneficial vegetable.

Soothing puffy eyes

One of the most common uses for cucumbers, other than eating them, is to soothe puffy eyes. Just cut two thick slices from a cold cucumber and place them over your closed eyes for 10 to 15 minutes to help reduce water retention. It's the ascorbic acid content (vitamin C) that helps to lessen eye puffiness almost instantly.

Create a brighter complexion with cucumber toner

A cucumber toner can help reduce skin puffiness, calm and tighten the skin and reveal a brighter complexion. You can use cucumber juice alone, or try this combination of ingredients:

½ cucumber (skin on), chopped
3 tablespoons witch hazel
2 tablespoons distilled water
Place all ingredients into a blender and blend until smooth. Pour the mix through a fine-mesh sieve to remove the solids and then pour the toner that remains into a clean bottle with a lid. Store it in the refrigerator and it will last several weeks.

Fade blemishes and acne scars

Just mix equal parts of cucumber juice and coconut water to fade skin blemishes and help whiten the skin. If you have acne scars, combine equal parts of lemon juice and cucumber juice to help fade or even remove them.

Preventing blemishes

An "anti-blemish" face mask can be made by blending a one-inch chunk of cucumber with one drop of rosemary essential oil and one egg white. Place the cucumber in a blender and blend until it turns to liquid, then add the drop of rosemary oil.

Whisk the egg white until it becomes stiff and fold it into the cucumber mixture. Apply to the face, avoiding the eye and mouth area. Allow it to sit for 15 minutes and then rinse off with a damp washcloth.

Treat combination skin

If you have combination skin (dry or normal in some areas, oily in others), use cucumber to create a mask that will help improve your complexion by mixing one half of a cucumber and one tablespoon of plain organic yogurt.

First puree the cucumber in a blender and then add the yogurt. Apply onto your face and neck and let it sit for about 20 minutes. Rinse with warm water followed by a splash of cold water.

Soothing sunburned skin

Cucumber is excellent for helping to soothe sunburned skin. If you were in the sun longer than you should have been, just apply cucumber juice to the affected area. It offers cooling and soothing effects and can also help to speed healing.

Fade dark circles

Rubbing cold cucumber slices under the eyes or applying cucumber juice can help to fade those annoying dark circles. Use a damp washcloth to remove after about 10 minutes. If you do this on a regular basis, your dark circles should start to fade gradually.

Make a cucumber salad

Eating cucumbers helps to improve skin from the inside out! Add some to a tossed baby spinach salad for a potent nutrition punch or make a salad base using chopped cucumbers mixed with fruits and other veggies.

The type of drinks you most avoid if you want to live long.

There are 3 harmful enemies living inside your kitchen. They're lurking in the darkness of your refrigerator right now... just sitting on the shelf, waiting for you to pour yourself another glass... and while you